What Do I Do?

How to Care for, Comfort,
and Commune With
Your Nursing Home Elder
(Revised and Illustrated Edition)

What Do I Do?
How to Care for, Comfort, and Commune With Your Nursing Home Elder

(Revised and Illustrated Edition)

By
Katherine Karr

Photographed by
Jesse Karr

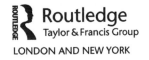
Routledge
Taylor & Francis Group
LONDON AND NEW YORK

What Do I Do? How to Care for, Comfort, and Commune With Your Nursing Home Elder (Revised and Illustrated Edition) has also been published as *Activities, Adaptation & Aging,* Volume 7, Number 1, September 1985.

First published 1985 by
The Haworth Press, Inc.

Published 2013 by Routledge
2 Park Square, Milton Park, Abingdon, Oxfordshire OX14 4RN
711 Third Avenue, New York, NY 10017, USA

First issued in paperback 2016

Routledge is an imprint of the Taylor & Francis Group, an informa business

Library of Congress Cataloging in Publication Data
Karr, Katherine.
   What do I do?

   Published also as v. 7, no. 1 of Activities, adaptation & aging.
   Includes bibliographical references.
   1. Geriatric nursing. 2. Aged—Care and hygiene. 1. Title.
RC954.3.K37 1985   613'.0438   85-7649

ISBN 13: 978-1-138-98704-3 (pbk)
ISBN 13: 978-0-86656-398-7 (hbk)

DEDICATED TO MY GRANDMOTHER, RUBY M. MILLER

Grandmother:

Your death gave to me new life and purpose.

Somehow I know you knew that would happen, and such was part of your having to end your life in a nursing home, rather than in the home you always made with your family.

You remain my teacher.

You remain my beloved.

What Do I Do?
How to Care for, Comfort, and Commune With Your Nursing Home Elder
(Revised and Illustrated Edition)

Activities, Adaptation & Aging
Volume 7, Number 1

CONTENTS

Acknowledgements

Special thanks are extended to Rest Harbor Nursing Home, Gresham, Oregon, and the Portland Adventist Convalescent Center, Portland, Oregon, for their cooperation in making the photography for this book possible.

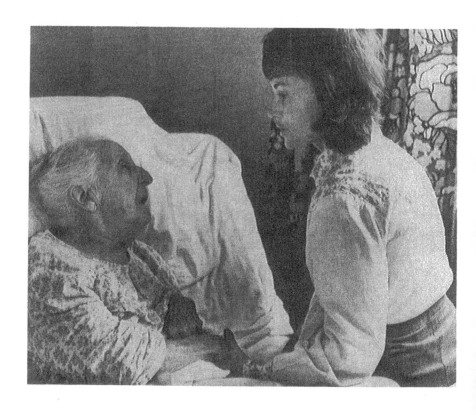

INTRODUCTION

WHAT *DO* YOU DO? For those who have known the closeness, comfort, and blessing of family involvement within either the closed or extended family circle, the placing of a family member in institutionalized care is an anguishing experience. Aside from the factors of guilt and anger, there comes a sense of loss that overwhelms. These personal factors are, of themselves, difficult with which to cope. But to them are added the needs of the family member now given over to the care of strangers. How to insure the same quality of care that family member has been accustomed to in his/her home setting becomes a concern of monumental proportions.

Faced with these painful matters, the most commonly asked question is: "How do I find a *good* nursing home, one which will administer sensitively to needs other than daily maintenance of my loved one?" For most, however, the question is untenable. Often the choice of nursing homes is restricted; either because many are filled to capacity at the time of the selection process, or considerations of cost and/or Medicaid limit one's choices. And all too often, quality care cannot be realistically assessed until one experiences it 24 hours a day, day in, day out. At most, it can be said that care givers reflect the continuum of care giving found throughout service and serving relationships: exemplary, passable, mediocre-to-poor.

As such, this book is *not* about the quality of care given or not given by nursing home facilities. Nor does it take as its premise that nursing homes *should* provide the kind of quality care family members provide for those of their own whom they cherish. Even the finest of institutional care lacks that special quality of love and sensitivity which only those in close, meaningful relationships of long-standing are able to extend to one another.

Instead, this book is written to encourage and guide family members and friends of institutionalized populations; family members and friends who understand that "quality care" is a function of "quality love". As such, it allows no limitations of institutional walls, is in no way diminished by the anguish of separation, nor finds acceptable the transfer of its responsibility to strangers.

That is not to imply such care giving is easy. Rather, it challenges us to the depths of our being. It can be time consuming, energy draining and stress producing. Simultaneously, it is comforting, confirming, and profoundly fulfilling.

This book is written in the hopes that the author's experiences in learning how to rise to those challenges may be of value to those in similar situations. For it was by answering the question: "WHAT DO I DO" that our family grew and deepened in love.

AN IMPENETRABLE REALITY FROM WHICH ALL STEREOTYPES SPRING: TOO OLD. TOO USELESS. TOO WORTHLESS. TOO BAD!

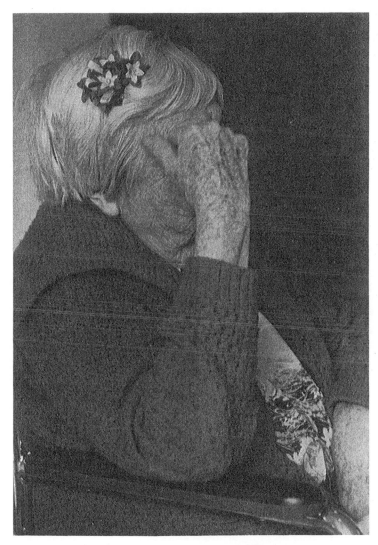

A REALITY THAT CHANGES WITH: REACHING OUT, REACHING TO. . . . .
No longer: "TOO OLD. TOO USELESS. TOO BAD." But rather,

"I'M HERE. I'M PRESENT BECAUSE OF YOUR PRESENCE."

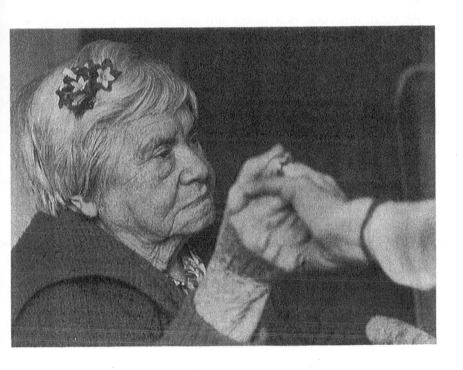

The message simple and obvious: the act of relationship gives greater meaning to life. Sometimes the physical act of touch is sufficient for communion with one's nursing home elder; other times sharing activities, memories, emotions or spiritual moments become the touchstone for meaningful interaction.

As such, this book is divided into four areas of care giving: physical, emotional, mental, and spiritual. Each section contains suggestions for caring, comforting, and communing in ways most needed by our nursing home elders.

HOW TO CARE FOR, COMFORT, AND COMMUNE AT THE PHYSICAL LEVEL

Care that reaches out from love, reaches out on all levels. Physically, it understands that a body lovingly groomed and cared for feels good inside and out,

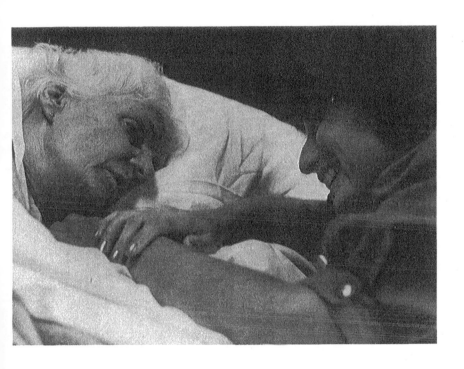

regardless of how infirm or bedridden a family member may be.

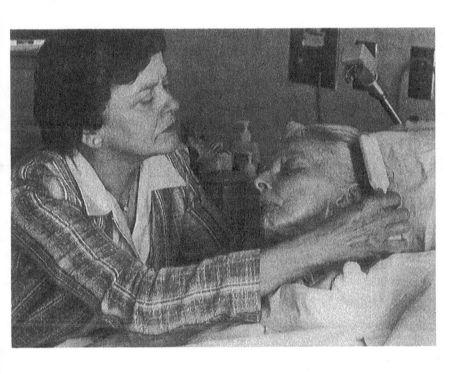

To be elderly, infirm, and institutionalized does not mean one has less need of grooming and loving attention. The need is all the greater.

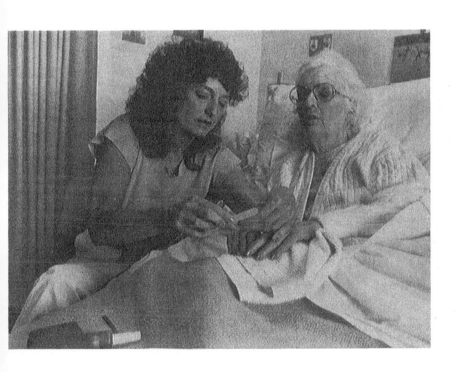

Take for example, massage. This is the kind of care that is of immeasurable help to the physical body. There probably is not a better way to express love while at the same time adding to the feeling of overall well being.

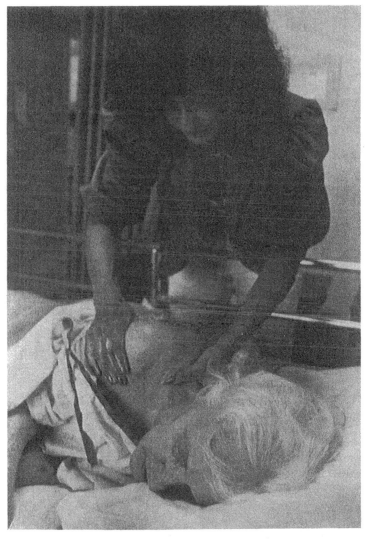

Massage nourishes the body by increasing blood flow to areas impaired by poor circulation. As important, however, is the nourishment it gives through touch; a form of comforting words cannot equal.

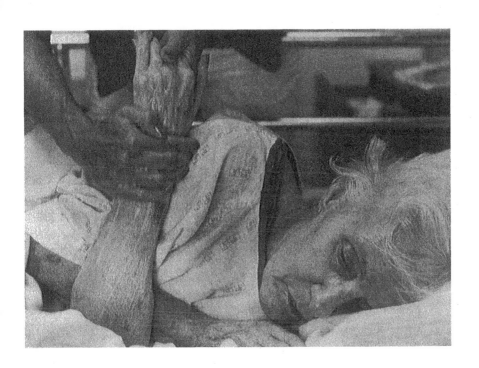

Family members that are committed to being an integral part
of their elder's care within the nursing home setting, are the
families that insure no needs go unmet.

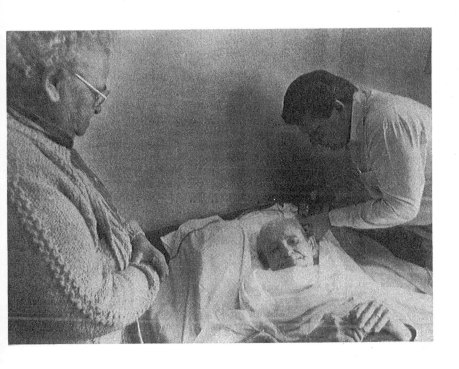

Besides, it feels better to have your haircut when the barber is your son!

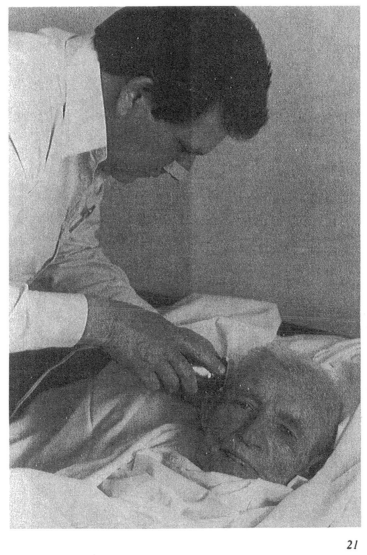

Mealtime is an important focal point for institutionalized elders. It is looked forward to for its opportunities of interaction, every bit as much as for its taste and nourishment.

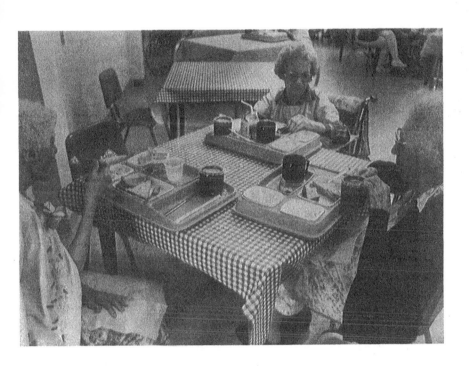

But many elders cannot feed themselves well; nor are they able to participate in the interaction of a dining room. Having a family member present to help them eat means they eat better and have a much more enjoyable time while eating.

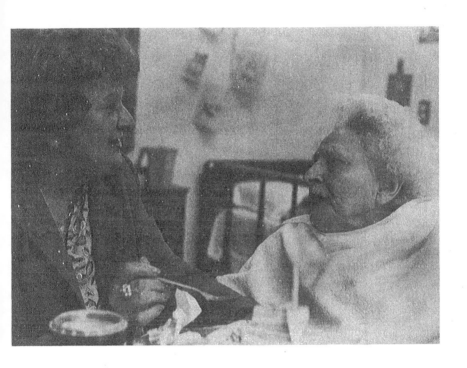

Most nursing homes have some kind of physical or restorative therapy conducted by professionally trained staff,

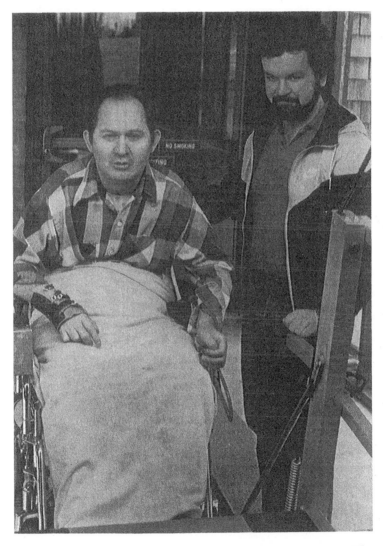

but getting outside with someone special is probably even more therapeutic.

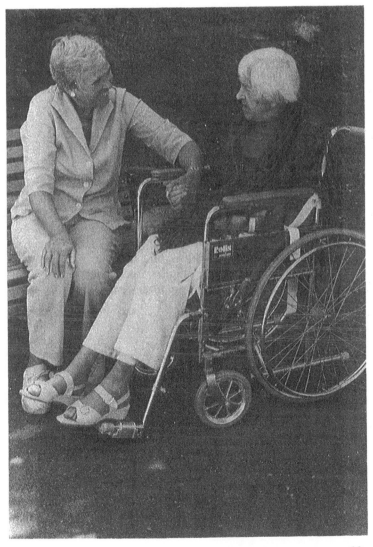

Proper nutrition, exercise, and grooming are all in the domain of physical well being. Yet, they give no guarantee. Neither do their administration by family members and friends. but in that act of outreach, lies a healing force that will never be packaged in pills.

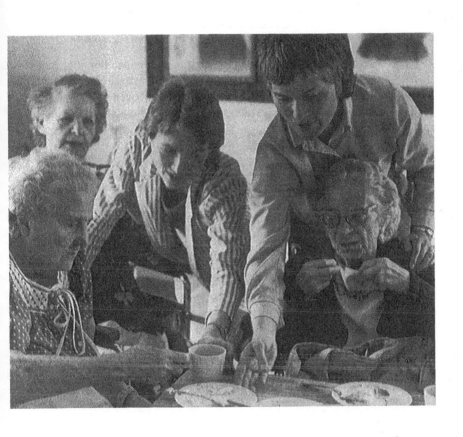

The guidelines that follow are suggestions for families helping care for their elder's physical needs.

CHECKPOINT:
CLOTHING NEEDS AND CLOTHING CARE

Laundry services are available in all homes, but that is
usually the extent of clothing care. This is an area that needs
close monitoring by family and friends, for even full closets
reveal items in varying states of disrepair and unuseability due
to neglect.

Concerns:

1. Institutional laundry can be extremely harsh on clothes.
   Buttons disappear, zippers come off tracks, seams split.
   Mending and repair services are not always a part of
   nursing home laundry services, and when they are, oversights are common.
2. Synthetic materials, although easier to handle in institutional laundry facilities, provide less warmth than cotton
   and wool blends. This is true in dresses and shirts and
   sleeping garments as well as hosiery. Older bodies are
   colder bodies, needing special warmth considerations.
3. Garments are often placed on residents backwards. If the
   person is incontinent or has stiffness or paralysis in the
   upper regions, it is easier for dressing and changing pur-
   poses to have dresses and robes open in the back with
   lower portions tucked alongside rather than under the
   resident. PROBLEM: Demeaning appearance; fit of
   clothing is awkward and uncomfortable, and the dignity
   of the person suffers considerably.
4. Knees and legs especially become cold when sitting hour
   after hour in a wheelchair. Coverings are necessary

which launder well. Two or three afghans are a minimum per person. Homes seldom provide more than one.

What Do I Do?

1. Periodically check all clothing, attending to needed repair work as identified. (Other elders in the room who don't have family to help minister to them could use assistance in this area also. It takes minimal time to sew on buttons and mend tears.)
   If feasible, consider doing your elder's laundry at home. Usually there will be a reduction in monthly costs, and the clothing will fare better.
2. Substitute cotton/wool stockings for nylon, especially in the fall and winter months. A variety of patterns, colors, and textures are available in long, warm hose. If poly-ester garments must make up the majority of the wardrobe, see that a supply of warm sweaters is on hand. Buy flannel nightgowns rather than synthetic sheerer blends, investing in the warmth and comfort of your elder at night.
3. Slit dresses, shirts and robes up the back; face, stitch velcro or hooks and eyes on the upper 10″ of the opening, sewing the front part of the garment closed. Cost factor: notions and time. Savings in dignity: immense.
4. Make certain two or three afghans or lap robes are available. Colorful ones add much in the way of brightness and pleasure.

Resources:

1. Fashion-Able Company: Rock Hill, New Jersey, 09553. Write for their catalogue (50ᶜ) containing numerous self-help items and a good selection of "easy on, easy off" clothing.

Vocational Guidance and Rehabilitation Service: 2239 E. 55th Street, Cleveland, Ohio 44103. Catalog available with clothing similarly designed for the elderly and disabled.
2. Check local department stores for nightgowns that open in the back (sometimes located in budget sections).
3. For Portland, Oregon, residents: GERI-FASHIONS: 777-4225; 3006 S.E. 81st, Portland. Lovely hand-made, nominally priced garments designed especially for nursing home residents—all with back openings.

CHECKPOINT:
SKIN CARE

The skin undergoes considerable change as one ages; it becomes more fragile and commences to break down. Lack of exercise and sunshine also present problems.

Concerns:

1. If the family member is incontinent, it is most critical to monitor closely the skin in the genital area. This is most easily done when the elder is in bed and can be turned for closer inspection.
2. If the family member is not incontinent, there still is a possibility that during the night they urinate in bed and are not cleaned until morning.
3. A major concern is the form of "learned incontinence" that is found in nursing homes. This is due to lack of available staff to help the elder to the bathroom or commode when they need to use it. Many are unable to use those facilities by themselves; that is one of the reasons they are in a nursing home.
4. In addition to the skin in the genital areas, the over-all

skin condition must be of on-going concern. Many of the impediments of the elderly (such as sluggish liver) contribute to dry skin. Lying or sitting in one unvariable position causes the skin to break down. Bruising is common.

What Do I Do?

1. Each and every visit check the condition of the skin.
2. Massage as much of the body as possible with creams and lotions. Pure unadulterated oils such as olive, almond, and safflower are lubricants which also nourish the skin; other lotions contain Vitamin E which is helpful.
3. Touch is therapeutic. Coupling touch with stroking, and rubbing warm lotions and oils is a special form of two-way communication. Our elders are the most isolated segment in the population, greatly deprived of physical contact.

   Pragmatically, caring for and nourishing the skin carries with it important physical benefits, but from an emotional standpoint, the benefits are equally as important. Often there is little one can actually *say* which helps an elder feel better, but massage and touch can be used to convey concern, care, and love.
4. Perform a simple experiment. One day simply sit and visit with your family member. The next visit, continue to share while you are creaming your elder's hands, massaging the arms, legs and feet with lotion. Notice the difference.
5. Most elders have impaired circulation. If they are wheelchair confined, remove their shoes and socks and notice any purple-bluish condition of the feet. If not a pronounced color change, most often the person will speak about their feet feeling cold. Be aware of the

change, however, when you massage their feet and legs, hands and arms. Circulation is *greatly* increased. It is hoped the day will come when massage is an integral part of health care, particularly for the bed ridden or wheel-chair confined individual. In the meanwhile, family and friends can administer to the skin care needs, improve circulation, and express love through touch.

CHECKPOINT:
OTHER PHYSICAL CONSIDERATIONS

Normally, this area should be a routine part of nursing services; families have found it wise, however, to check these areas as well.

Concerns:

1. Kidney, bladder and prostate diseases are found with advancing years. The decrease in circulation of blood through the kidneys can cause uremia; uremia can also occur in conditions of dehydration when the elder's body is depleted of water, such as happens after vomiting or with diarrhea or during fevers. It can also be brought on by certain drugs.
2. Constipation is a stubborn problem for many residents, particularly for those bedridden. Many require some bowel aid, but it is wise not to use harsh laxatives. Natural stool softeners can help avoid painful fecal impactions which occur when putty-like accumulations of waste material collect in the rectum.
3. Complaints of a diminishing sense of taste or of a bitter, perhaps sour taste or of a dry tongue are not unusual among elders. Some changes in taste perception are caused by breathing through the mouth. However, cer-

tain medications can cause dryness of the mouth and/or bitter tastes; these are medications like digitalis, belladonna-like drugs, or those used in rheumatic disorders.

4. "Wrist drop" may occur when an elder rests arms or wrists too long on the arms of a chair. The continued pressure over the nerves at the elbows or palm side of the forearms creates the limpness, making the wrists drop.

5. "Side-tilt" occurs when the body seems to tilt or fall over the side of a wheel chair. The elder lolls over one arm of the chair, with body completely off balance from erect sitting position.

6. "Edema" which is a puffiness in the legs and ankles may develop when an elder spends most of his/her day sitting in one position.

7. Bed pan elders may be powdered but not wiped or washed after urinating. The same may hold true for those using commodes. Redness or rash developing in the genital areas would indicate this is the case.

What Do I Do?

1. Kidney infections often cause pain in the small of the back, with the elder experiencing irritation of the bladder, burning and frequent urination; perhaps scanty urination. If kidney/bladder problems are suspected, request a urinalysis to determine the nature of the cause.

2. Check your elder's daily bowel and bladder records twice or three times a week. If s/he is not eating well, complains of abdominal pain or is distended in the intestinal area, have nursing staff check for impaction. Impaction may not be detected by changing staff unless nursing assistants are assigned to the same residents and are alert to the day-to-day elimination schedules.

3. Parsley or mint teas help sweeten breath; also soothe digestion. Mints or enzyme preparations may help the

bitter or sour tastes. Check the medications in use to determine if they are necessary if they cause these side-effects.

4. "Wrist drop", "Side tilt", and "Edema" are concerns which may be due to position rather than disease. In the case of wrist drop, soft cushions on the chair can help alleviate.

5. Side tilt can be corrected through the use of small pillows placed in back of shoulders and along the side of the elder to counter the tilt and help prop the body back into a vertical position. Sometimes it is more comfortable to roll a small blanket or afghan for the added support.

6. Edema may be helped by frequent changes in position. Restorative therapy exercising limbs by moving them gently horizontally and vertically in the wheelchair is of considerable benefit.

7. Continued oversights in personal care are an administrative problem and should be called to the attention of those in charge.

CHECKPOINT:
TEETH AND DENTURE CARE

This is a crucial area, since neglected mouths eventually are unable to chew and enjoy food.

Concerns:

There is a great lack of dental care in nursing homes in the sense of periodic, regular check-ups and cleaning by professionally trained persons. Dentures are often broken or lost.

What Do I Do?

1. Dentures must be marked, so if misplaced, they will be returned to their proper owner.

2. Check continually the condition of dentures and teeth. Be prepared to subject them to thorough cleansings and brushings.
3. Make sure dentures are being soaked nightly and that there are adequate supplies of denture cleanser on hand. (Denture cleanser disappears rapidly if used for other residents whose supplies have been depleted.)
4. Determine if there are community service or social service programs in your area wherein dentists give volunteer hours to work with nursing homes. Are there community programs that might be receptive to sponsoring such a program? (In Portland, Oregon, grant monies have made it possible for dentistry school personnel to work with nursing homes who are willing to share the costs.)

CHECKPOINT:
EYE CARE

Eyesight, like hearing, is essential to one's sense of well being. Acuity diminishes as one ages, glaucoma and cataracts become more prevalent.

Concerns:

Prescriptions tend not to be changed once an elder enters a nursing home; seldom are the eyes checked of those who have not worn glasses to-date. Glasses become lost or broken, frames need adjustment because of all the handling they receive by different personnel in the home, as well as by the owner.

What Do I Do?

1. Make certain glasses are clearly labeled so they can be returned to their owner if misplaced.
2. If possible, take your family member periodically to your

family optometrist/ophthalmologist to have their eyes tested and frames adjusted. This is especially important if the nursing home has no professional visiting to check each resident.

3. Determine if there are local community groups that would like to upgrade eye care in nursing homes. The Lions, a national service group, have an international commitment to vision. (One Lion's group in Portland, Oregon, has developed an eye program with local nursing homes in their area of the city in conjunction with students from the optometry program of a near-by college. This kind of outreach needs to be encouraged. People helping people!)

CHECKPOINT:
EAR CARE

Because hearing is basic to one's sense of well-being, this becomes a vital area of concern.

Concerns:

It is said that much of the seeming deafness in the elderly is more related to wax build-up than actual nerve or tone deafness. However, ear care is less apt to be checked in bathing or routine care needs than other bodily parts. Since hearing does tend to become progressively less acute as years pass, when is there a place for a hearing aid, and if one is being worn, how functional is it?

What Do I Do?

1. Cleaning and oiling of the ears needs to be done on a regular schedule. This will not remove the more deeply plugged wax pockets if they exist, but it will keep interference wax to a minimum.

2. Residential facilities all have off-premise physicians whose designated job is to periodically visit each patient and check on their condition. Request ear examinations as part of the visit. If embedded wax is suspected, it can be removed under the physician's supervision. The customary procedure is to apply two drops of baby oil, mineral oil or glycerin in the ear at night for three days. After the third night, the ears are flushed with a small rubber bulb syringe, using warm water with distilled vinegar.

3. Batteries on hearing aids need to be serviced periodically. Seldom will hearing aids be checked by staff. They need to be cleaned regularly, because ear wax collects in and around them.

CHECKPOINT:
HAIR GROOMING AND COSMETOLOGY NEEDS

Beauticians usually affiliate with nursing homes on a part-time basis. There is an additional charge for their services. If you cannot include this cost for your elder, or if a beautician is not available, shampoos will be given as part of the shower/bathing process.

Concerns:

Hair allowed to drip-dry results in cold susceptibility; it is also uncomfortable. Nursing assistants may not have sufficient time to comb and style hair. Regular brushing and scalp massage is seldom possible.

What Do I Do?

1. Determine the shampoo/shower schedule. Arrange to be there to dry family member's hair, taking along a portable dryer if necessary.

Encourage facility to purchase portable hair dryers if not presently available. They are needed in addition to a stationary one.

2. Combing and brushing the hair is an excellent way of stimulating far more than hair follicles. Such stroking is therapeutic, bringing blood to surface areas of the brain. Elders enjoy the feeling; it is a special way of making contact.

CHECKPOINT:
NAILS—MANICURING AND PEDICURING

Older bodies are generally not flexible enough to bend down to care for toes; nor do older hands easily wield nail scissors. Both toes and fingers can ache and become less easily manipulated if nails are neglected.

Concern:

Podiatrists tend to be scheduled infrequently in homes, if at all. Nursing assistants may not have directives to administer to this area of need. Further, it is much easier on the residents to have hands and feet soaked first prior to trimming the nails. Seldom does staff have time free for this.

What Do I Do?

1. Plan a monthly period expressly for pedicures. This is more easily done with two persons, since feet need to be soaked first in warm water before trimming, and that is awkward in a wheel chair. This is also an appropriate time for cleaning and oiling the skin in the areas between the toes not readily accessible.
2. Keep nail scissors, file, and emery boards with you each

time you visit so immediate manicuring needs can be handled on the spot. However, as with toenails, there is still a place for setting aside special periods for oiling cuticles and administering to special cleaning, clipping needs.

CHECKPOINT: BEDSORES

Bedsores occur when continuous pressure against beds or wheelchairs causes ulceration. They tend to occur on the lower spine, side of the hips, and on heels, although they can be found any place on the body.

Concerns:

If your elder's skin has commenced to break down and/or if they can no longer walk and are confined to a wheelchair or bed, this is a key area to monitor. Any or all of the following factors can contribute to bedsores:

1. Remaining in one position for too long (bed or chair, especially when there is pressure on a particular area);
2. Wrinkled bed clothing;
3. Lack of cleanliness from causes such as soiling or excessive perspiration;
4. Inadequate food intake or inadequate nourishment which inhibits the body's natural repair function;
5. Poor circulation.

What Do I Do?

1. Make sure your elder is turned often so as to prevent prolonged pressure on any one part of the body.

2. Give special attention to the areas of the lower back, hips or heels if discoloration should appear. The first evidence of bedsores beginning to form is a pink or reddish surface over a pressure area. Should that be the case, make sure your elder lies in a position wherein pressure is minimized. Alert staff and request conference with the director of nursing.
3. Special devices are designed to keep pressure off discolored skin and bedsores. They are known as rubber or foam "donuts", and are available at most drugstores. They somewhat resemble dry floats children use in learning to swim.
4. Lambskins are very soft and allow the air to circulate next to the skin. Large foam mattress mats have been designed expressly to prevent bedsores and are available through hospital supply houses if there is no access through the nursing home.
5. No one method may be entirely satisfactory. Obtain the advice of the professional staff. However, cleanliness and freedom from pressure are the most important factors in the prevention and cure of bedsores.

CHECKPOINT: MONITORING MEDICATIONS

Nursing home residents as a population are over-medicated. Statistics are alarming in this area.

Concerns:

Over $500 million dollars are spent yearly on nursing home drugs; tranquilizers constitute 20% of that total. There is a growing realization that in the elderly, drugs may have especially toxic and undesirable reactions because of elders' reduced metabolic activity and altered central nervous system reaction. Drugs are frequently administered in ignorance of the unique biochemical and psychological make-up of the elderly person, as well as in ignorance of the food which is incompatible with such medications.

The number and frequency of interactions and side effects for a predominance of drugs increases with age. Drugs taken concurrently may nullify one another, escalate harsh and unexpected results. The average age of nursing home residents is 82. Their average pharmacological intake is between five and seven different drugs daily; some taken twice or three times.

What Do I Do?

1. The most common medications which are over-prescribed are the tranquilizer/sedative group. Frequently they are ordered at the urging of the nursing home staff, since a tranquilized elder is much quieter than one who is boisterous. Many such medications are prescribed by an M.D. on a "PRN" basis (as necessary) which allows the local staff autonomy in deciding when use is required. Request a conference with the director of nursing and administrators if you suspect this is the case with your elder. As a family member, you have legal access to daily medication records and may check to see what is being administered and when.
2. A related problem arises with medications that are prescribed and not stopped when the concern is resolved. It is critical to review regularly the medications prescribed, and determine if there are those which can be discontinued. The time and trouble often needed for up-dating needs can mean the difference between whether your elder is alert and vibrant or sleepy and dull.
3. Learn to use the *Physician's Desk Reference Guide* (PDR), a sourcebook wherein all medications are listed,

giving the known side effects for each and every drug on the market. Most libraries have this publication in their Reference Section. Not only with the PDR give you information on what to look for regarding the side-effects of the drug, it may lead you to question whether the gain from administration is worth the price paid elsewhere by the body.

CHECKPOINT:
DIETARY AWARENESS

Meals are often the most awaited part of the day in a nursing home. However, there are vast differences in quality and quantity of food.

Concerns:

1. Nursing home food services tend not to provide fresh fruits and vegetables; the majority are canned, some frozen. Meals can succumb to the typical institutional failing: too much starch, too much salt, too much sugar, too many processed, adulterated foods. Important vitamins and minerals are often missing or lost through overcooking or resting on steam tables.
2. The average total cost per day to cover all three meals per elder is $1.50 (1979 statistics).
3. Institutional food can be a dramatic change from the kind of diet your elder has been accustomed to over the years.
4. Water must be easily available 24 hours. The role of fluids in flushing the sedentary system is critical. Water pitchers may be on hand but many elders forget to drink unless encouraged throughout the day.

What Do I Do?

1. Vitamin deficiencies are recognizable by any one or combination of the following: excessively dry skin, lack of energy, slick red tongue, over-sensitivity to sunlight, cracks at the corners of the mouth, poor night vision. If any of these occur, or you have grounds for feeling the diet is not a balanced one nutritionally, include daily vitamin/mineral supplements.

   If your elder becomes exhausted for no apparent reason, check for anemia. Although one cause may be bleeding from the bowel, a second primary cause is directly related to a diet deficient in fresh meat and leafy green vegetables. Alert your physician and the nursing staff if you suspect anemia.

2. If you are concerned about the quality of food or the lack of it, request your physician to order a special diet: i.e. one consisting of fresh fruits and vegetables, high protein or whatever else you feel is lacking. These orders must be complied with if the elder is receiving State aid.

3. Bring foods from home to supplement the institutional food. Undoubtedly your elder has food preferences. Making those preferences available when possible is a special form of caring. Some foods admittedly create problems, such as ripe juicy fruit. Seedless green grapes would be a better choice than overripe peaches.

   Ice cream, favorite beverages, flavorful soups can be conveniently carried in thermos bottles. Visit during meal times so you can find out the kind and quality of food being served. It is instructional to do this for breakfast as well as the later meals.

4. If water is not immediately available and changed daily, request a change in policy. Encourage your elder to drink often. Work with staff so they will give continual re-

minders if such is necessary. Juices are usually served at least twice a day. However, a glass may go unnoticed or hands may be unable to guide it to lips unaided.

CHECKPOINT:
SPECIAL FEEDING CONSIDERATIONS

Your elder may reach a time wherein s/he has difficulty swallowing or chewing. The time may come when they cannot feed themselves or when they refuse all food.

Concerns:

1. Elders who have to be fed by nursing assistants are often rushed because of time schedules. Difficulties eating can necessitate 20-30 minutes for an adequate feeding. This is not possible for an assistant who has another four or five elders to feed.
2. When special care is required for the feeding process, short staff or those insensitive or indifferent can complicate the situation. Blasé or non-communicative feeding reduces the meal to a mechanical act with dehumanizing overtones.

What Do I Do?

1. Try to have family coverage for one meal every day. Meals are meant to be times for sharing, caring and enjoying communion. Family members will have the sensitivity to the needs of the elder that staff may lack. The elder will not be hurried if a family member is in charge of the feeding process.
2. If your elder cannot swallow solid food, they will be placed on a liquid form of diet. Their food will be

pureed; soups will be an integral part of meals. The family may feel the need to supplement, particularly if they have no knowledge of what is being injested. Pureed baby food can be bought in jars of a wide variety. A number of high protein drinks are available, ranging from powders found in health and natural food stores to those of supermarket variety (the latter having a somewhat higher sugar and sodium content). These can be prepared at home and carried to the facility in thermos bottles.

If spoon feeding is too tedious with very little being swallowed, use straws. If they are ineffective, ask the staff to place the pureed food or liquid in a syringe. Care must be taken in this process, and it is recommended that the nursing staff supervise.

There are always those times when it is better not to force feed. If your elder is choosing not to eat (consciously or unconsciously) and even refuses special preparations from home, such is their choice. From our vantage point, they may seem to be out-of-contact to make such a decision, but the body has its own inherent wisdom, and if it desires minimal or no food as it prepares for another journey, such wishes should be honored.

CHECKPOINT:
RESTORATIVE THERAPY

This is a term used to designate physical therapy so the body may regain flexibility or remain functioning more fully.

Concerns:

Some homes have restorative therapy available to residents; others do not. Even if the program is comprehensive, it may be for only a short period three or four times a week. There is always the need to supplement it on the part of a family member when possible.

What Do I Do?

1. If your family member is able to receive restorative therapy, spend time with the restorative aides to find out the extent of the program designed for him/her. Draw on their expertise to learn ways you can work on your own to compliment their program. That may take the form of exercises, walking, finger, arm and leg manipulations. A visiting period is an ideal time to assist in these areas.

2. Physical exercises geared to the capacity and age of your elder are a meaningful, yet most practical way of caring and sharing. Some suggestions to begin with:

   Ball throwing. "Nerf" balls are ideal for playing catch. They are soft, light and pliable. This type of activity can be done easily with one confined to a wheel chair. It provides stimulation, helps keep hands and fingers flexible, is a source of joy and laughter, and gives a sense of accomplishment.

   Clapping hands, touching shoulders, touching eyes, touching ears, touching knees—all to the beat of a clap—keeps hands and body in use and is a good way of encouraging self-stimulation for one in a wheelchair.

   Bean bags, silly putty, latch hooking all lend themselves to restorative therapy. Craft work through the activities program aids in this area, particularly if a family member can join in, adding encouragement for finger and hand motion.

HOW TO CARE FOR, COMFORT, AND COMMUNE AT THE EMOTIONAL LEVEL

Emotional needs are among the most powerful needs of institutionalized populations. Removed from family and community, it is difficult to believe one is still worthwhile and loved unless families convey that affirmation through regular visits.

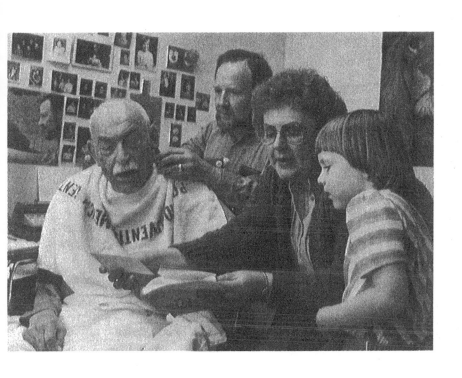

Much time is spent alone when living in a nursing home. It is the aloneness that comes with loss of one's roots; the aloneness that arises when dependence replaces independence.

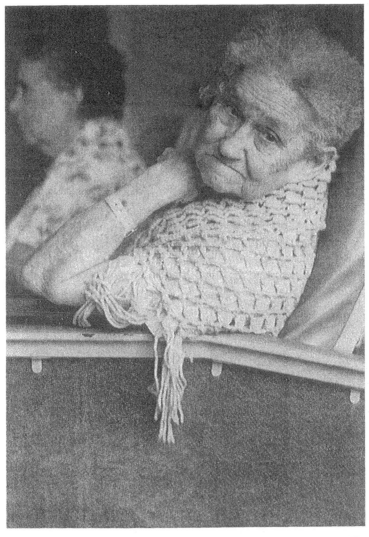

It is often difficult for family members to respond to their elder's emotional pain because problem solving is not possible. The elder cannot go home; nor will they regain their independence.

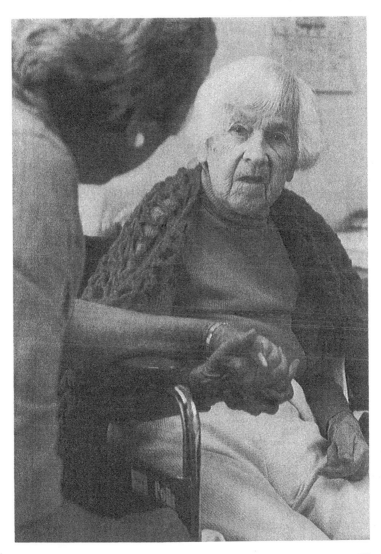

In the face of such emotional tearings, touch is the one genuine response. Touch communicates an understanding that is not rendered awkward by words.

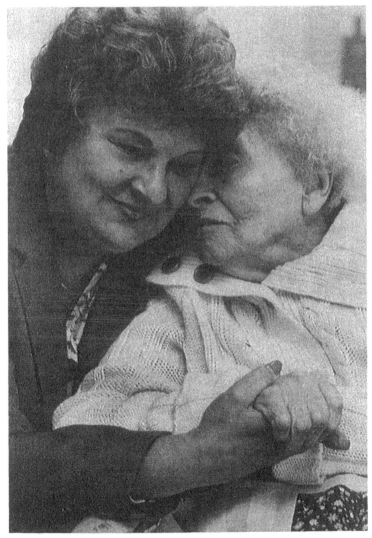

Pets are increasingly being acknowledged for their role in satisfying otherwise unmet emotional needs. Fragile elders are among the most touch hungry of persons. A warm, furry friend both feels good and spreads joy.

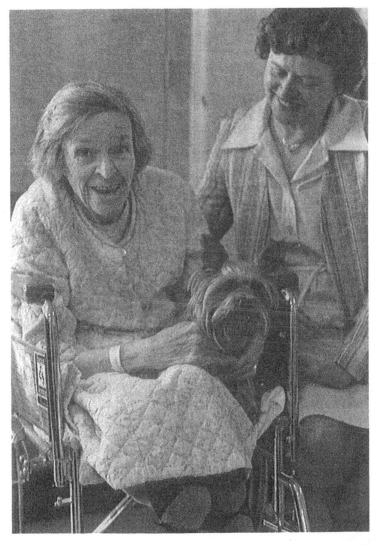

But animals can never replace the tenderness of human inter-action. Animals have their special place, but needed most is the warm, caressing care expressed person-to-person.

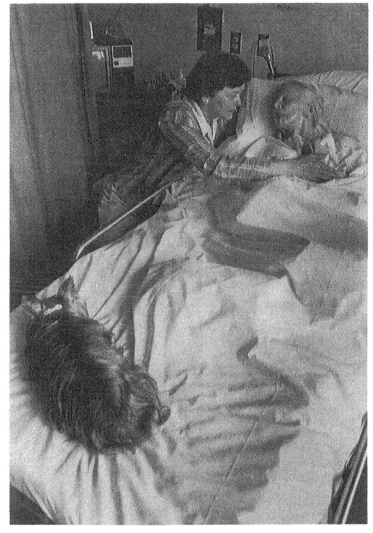

That care is especially appreciated at seasonal holidays and birthdays. And if the elder cannot be taken home to share in the event, then families can bring the celebration to their elder.

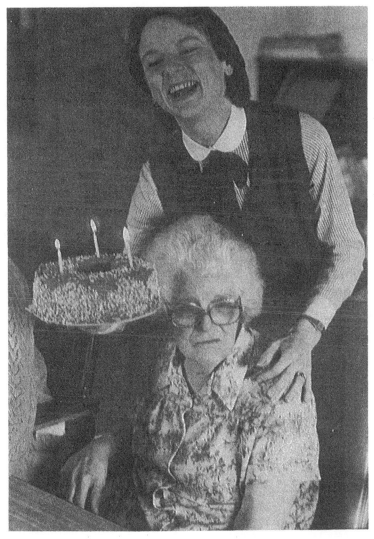

Few of us are adequately schooled in the expression of emotion. Communication skills in this area can be learned, but skills can never replace spontaneous child-like emotional interaction with those we love.

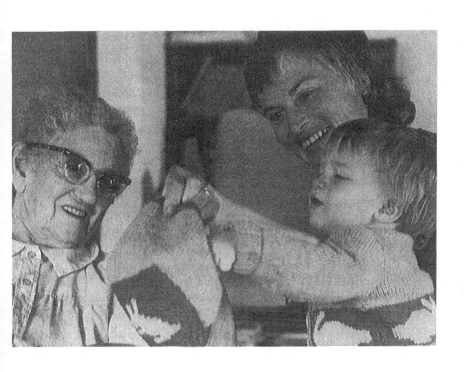

The guidelines that follow are for families caring for their elder's emotional needs.

CHECKPOINT:
UNDERSTANDING FEELINGS
AND DEVELOPING EMPATHY SKILLS

The cause most commonly cited for the loneliness and growing withdrawal in the nursing home environment is that of having no one to talk with or one who is willing to listen. Some of this concern can be addressed by upgrading activities programs and mental kinds of stimulation (see next section). However, in the emotional realm, family members can help combat loneliness and withdrawal by cultivating empathy and active listening skills.

Concerns:

Nursing home employees are not trained in psychological skills; nor is such a part of their job description. It calls for an investment of time and energy to listen and respond to the emotional needs of elders. Seldom is this kind of time available. Moreover, physical care takes priority over emotional care by the nature and structure of nursing homes.

What Do I Do?

1. Be aware of the need for *empathy* when spending time with elders. Empathy is the nonjudgemental awareness that helps the other person know you understand and accept their feelings. Empathy is akin to being inside the other person's skin and experiencing the world through their eyes, body and mind-set.

2. Most often people are very judgemental about others' emotional states, particularly the more negative ones. Messages are sent out such as: "You shouldn't be angry", "Don't be so upset, you know they are doing the best they can", "Snap out of your depression; you are just feeling sorry for yourself."

Those kinds of messages are basically telling the other person their feelings are not legitimate and they should somehow be different from what and who they are. Messages like those hurt and make matters worse.

Empathy, on the other hand, realizes the feeling *is* legitimate and accepts it rather than encouraging the other to change. In so doing, the unique personhood of the other has been acknowledged; he or she feels understood, and the concern is not as weighty as when carried alone.

3. Following are examples of a situation wherein emotions are handled first unskillfully and them empathetically.

"Oh Mother, I get so tired of your complaining. What do you mean you are lonely and don't get good care here? You have a nice room and enjoy your food. You have everything you need, and it's just ridiculous to sit there and cry. You just want attention, that's all." (Family member leaves frustrated and mad.)

"Mother, I know it is difficult to be in a place you are not used to. I realize there is not a lot for you to do and that your roommate isn't able to visit with you very much. It must be very lonely when you are not able to see your family and friends as much as you would like, and even though you have a nice room and good food, that really doesn't make up for it, does it? I feel so bad when I see you sitting there crying because I don't know what to do. I love you so much and wish you didn't have to be here either." (Family member pulls chair closer and sits holding elder, conveying comfort through silent touch.)

CHECKPOINT:
USING TOUCH TO COMMUNICATE CARE

Touch is magic; mysterious because it is so powerful; necessary for life. Babies can die of a disease called marasmus if they are not held, stroked, and fondled. One never outgrows their need for touch. Unfortunately, after childhood, words tend to substitute for this form of contact.

Concerns:

Institutional care is impersonal care by and large. Touch is reserved for bathing, dressing, feeding and the administration of medication. Nurses and nursing assistants do not have the time nor directives to give meaningful touch to residents.

What Do I Do?

1. Understanding the different forms of touch:
   Spontaneous forms: hugs, warm embraces, holding hands, caressing in your own special way.
   Pragmatic forms: foot and hand massage, brushing hair, creaming and oiling the skin, particularly the hands, arms, legs, and feet.
   Silent touch: Patter and chatter are often used to mask feelings of inadequacy and uncomfortableness. But like all other feelings, these are legitimate. Rather than attempt to repress them, better to acknowledge the awkwardness and talk about it in a non-judgemental fashion. Inevitably there is a real understanding on the part of the family member. Then to sit in quiet acceptance of one another's humanness, touching or holding hands, is a very special form of caring.
2. Understanding the different expressions of touch:
   The touch of comfort: This form of touch conveys: "I

feel with you and I want you to know I am here." Sometimes this may take the form of silent communication; other times it may be administering to the comfort needs via the pragmatic forms of caring touch.

The touch of love: This form of touch conveys: "I cherish you and want to be with you." Kisses, hugs, embraces, holding, stroking, and caressing all convey this type of love.

The touch of healing (known increasingly as "Therapeutic touch"): Seers have taught that our hands are for heeling, serving and blessing. There is now a movement in the nursing profession working with therapeutic touch. Although some skills may be important, and one may wish to read the literature, all of us have a natural ability to use our hands to comfort those in pain. Hands know what to do if we will listen and be guided by them. Massage skills can be useful in this regard.

The touch of anger, rejection or control: This form of touch basically says: "I resent you", "I want to change you or force you to do things my way". Touch can be as painful as it is loving; toxic as well as therapeutic. Any awareness of this kind of touch should be reported to administration when witnessed. Elders are entitled to only the most caring of touch.

3. The importance of touch:

One of the beauties of touch is that it produces a bodily reaction which is always more powerful than a mental reaction. When one is touched, he/she is touched in the body; it can be located and felt.

Touch is also reciprocal. When one sends out a message of love, concern (or resentment or anger), there is always a message received in return. It may be reinforcing: i.e. the touch of love being met with smiles and appreciation. But it also may be depreciating: i.e. a touch of love being met with stony silence or annoyance.

If the latter, it is important to keep in mind that many persons in our culture are not used to being touched; others have learned to avoid it. There may be a need to approach this area with caution, even with a loved family member. If so, the best and safest place to start is with the hands, simply holding or stroking gently.

Resources:

Kreiger, Delores: *Therapeutic Touch* (See bibliography)
Luce, Gay: *Your Second Life* (See bibliography)

CHECKPOINT:
OVERCOMING DISCOUNTING BEHAVIORS

A discount is a subtle way of putting another person down either by ignoring them or by implying what they say or do is not important. Discounts can be verbal or conveyed by facial expression, tone of voice or posture.

Concerns:

Institutional life all too often and all too mistakenly conveys second class citizenship. There is a tendency to treat elders like children, not taking their conversation or needs seriously. Prevalent forms of discounting: staff addressing residents by first names; staff discounting requests.
Example:
"May I wear my blue dress today?"
"You know you spill food over everything; you'll just get it dirty before your family comes."
Discounts basically say: *You don't count.*

What Do I Do?

1. Look first at own behaviors. It is always easier to see discounting behaviors in others.

2. Determine what kind of training skills are provided as part of in-service classes for staff members. Physical care needs are stressed, but so should psychological needs, particularly since so many physical ills are related to emotional concerns.
   Persons do not inherit sensitive and well-developed communication skills. Those who do not discount others are those who have learned why such behaviors are non-productive, disrespectful and non-growth producing. Communication skills are not yet taught in most schools; all the more reason to strengthen this area through in-service programs, seminars and workshops sponsored by nursing homes and other concerned parties.
3. It is said we teach primarily by our being. If communication skills are not being taught to staff members, then teach yourself through example. Love is not taught; it is caught. The same dynamic operates when persons have an opportunity to see caring behaviors in action.

CHECKPOINT:
PATRONIZING BEHAVIORS

Patronizing behaviors are a special form of discount wherein the elderly person is treated not with the dignity of his/her person, but as though they were children.

Concerns:

Patronizing behaviors run the full scale from baby-talking to over solicitous behavior, insincere flattery and fondling.
Prevalent patronizing behaviors: Wide use of infantilizing while caring, feeding and dressing the residents.
Example: ''Come on baby doll, just finish this last bitty sip of juicey for me.'' Hugging and fondling while exclaiming: ''Don't we look pretty today.''

What Do I Do?

1. As with discounting behaviors, first examine self and see if changes are in order.
2. Request in-service training programs so staff can appreciate how demeaning such actions are and how they reinforce childish behavior from elders.

CHECKPOINT:
THE ROLE OF MUSIC IN CARING

The healing, therapeutic value of music has been recognized from the earliest of times. It is a universal language that vibrates to one's innermost depths, creating a stronger, more joyful life force.

Concerns:

Television is the primary media form available in most nursing homes. Often it is watched simply to pass time since programs of an uplifting nature are few. Activities programs generally include some form of music, group singing or outside entertainers. However, these times are all too brief. Further, there are always those elders who may not be able to attend.

What Do I Do?

1. Bring music *to* your elder. Cassette players are widely available; prices are within the reach of most. Stores have good selection of tapes, making it easy to find those particularly enjoyed by your elder. If you have the appropriate outlets, it is not difficult to create your own tapes from the records you know your elder has enjoyed. Most states make available free use of cassettes and

record players. Check with the Family Services Division.

In lieu of cassettes, portable phonographs can accompany your visit. They are more cumbersome than cassettes but can be set up and favorite albums enjoyed in that fashion.

2. If family members play instruments or sing, how joyous to have that talent shared in the context of the nursing home. Most facilities have a piano easily accessible when planned activities are not in progress. Impromptu sing-alongs are often the most enjoyed. All it takes is a willingness to share one's talent with others. Nor does it have to be polished talent, as nursing home audiences are the most appreciative and least demanding in the community.

CHECKPOINT:
SPECIAL SEASONAL CONSIDERATIONS

Holidays can be a pleasure or a source of emotional pain depending upon how they are planned. The times families most want their elder with them are Christmas, Thanksgiving, Easter, birthdays, Mother's Day/Father's Day.

Concern:

No celebration, no matter how thoughtfully planned by a nursing home can replace family gatherings. Often on holidays, homes are short staffed which makes the day even less pleasant than one would hope.

What Do I Do?

1. When possible, make arrangements to bring your elder home to share in the family festivities. This requires ad-

vance planning and shaping the day around the special considerations of the infirm family member. That is more easily accomplished when there are other relatives and family members on hand, since three pairs of strong arms may be required for lifting, putting to bed, etc. (If family cannot transport, there is the additional cost of wheelchair transport. Those services get booked days and weeks before seasonal holidays so there is a need to plan early.)

2. If the family member cannot come home for the celebration, consider bringing home to the elder. Arrangements can be made with administration and dining room staff to have a family dinner on the premises at a time when the dining hall or recreation hall are not being used for residential activities. A special dinner or lunch can be "picnicked" in and shared in the context of the entire family, complete with presents, favors, and camera to capture the event.

HOW TO CARE FOR,
COMFORT,
AND COMMUNE
AT THE MENTAL LEVEL

Stimulation is the crucial factor in determining whether an institutionalized elder will continue to remain mentally alert.

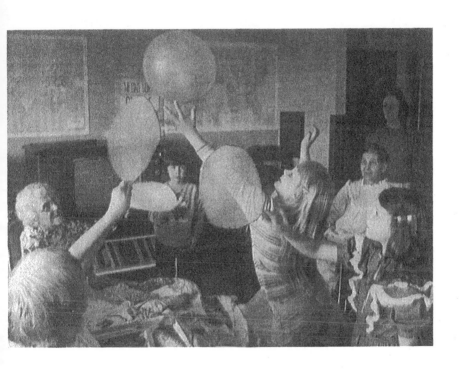

Activities programs in nursing homes have been designed to encourage that kind of stimulation.

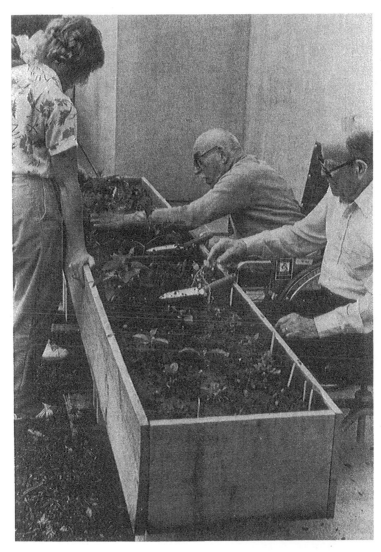

These need to be activities which are creative and challenging, rather than those which are diversionary, patronizing, and infantalizing.

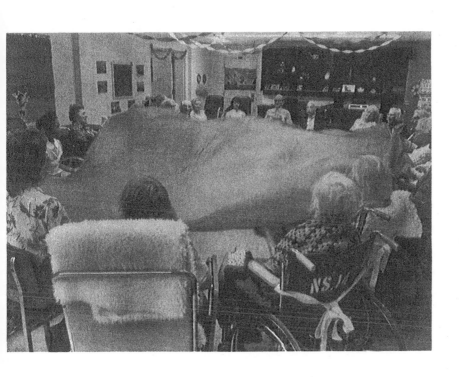

Real stimulation is joyful and affirming.

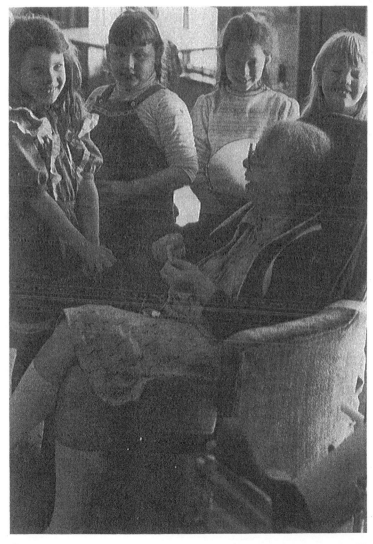

Composing poetry is a case in point. This is one of the most useful kinds of activities because it fosters mental stimulation as well as interaction among elders, affirming that what they have inside them is worthwhile.

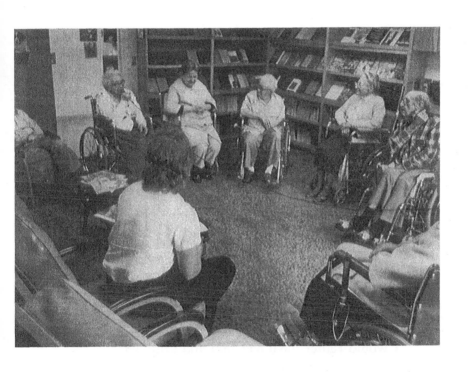

A POEM TO OUR GRANDMOTHER GOOSEBERRY

What I want to say to Grandmother Gooseberry
    I can't say in the parlour.

What I want to say to Grandmother Gooseberry
    Is that I could find a better name than that.

What I want to say to Grandmother Gooseberry
    Is God bless her and God bless gooseberries.
    We are supposed to pray for the wicked and the wild.

What I want to say to Grandmother Gooseberry
    Is that we need to pick more gooseberries
    And get more grandmothers.

                —Group poem composed by
                a nursing home poetry group
                conducted by the author.

BREAKFAST

It wasn't much of a breakfast.
It made a big lump in my stomach.
I would rather have had jam and crumpets.
Back home in Massachusetts, that's what we ate.
There I felt on top of the world.
Here I felt let down.

                —Blanche Lockwood

YOU BETTER KNOW ABOUT BUTTER

You better know about butter
because most of it today
sits on store shelves
like it grows there.
It don't.

When I was a girl
we churned our butter
straight out of the cow.
Well, not really.
It had to clabber first.
That's the secret of good butter.
If it clabbers up
too hot or too cold,
it's only fit for buttermilk.
But even your own buttermilk
was smacking good to drink.

Sometimes I got my hands cracked
because I sneaked the cream
before it could be used for butter.
But that way, my hands
didn't hurt near as much
as they did when it was my turn
to churn and churn and churn.
It always seemed like my arms
was going to fall
right into the butter.
There would have been
a licking for you.

—Ethel Schiedel

Poetry also provides the opportunity for residents to express inner feelings:

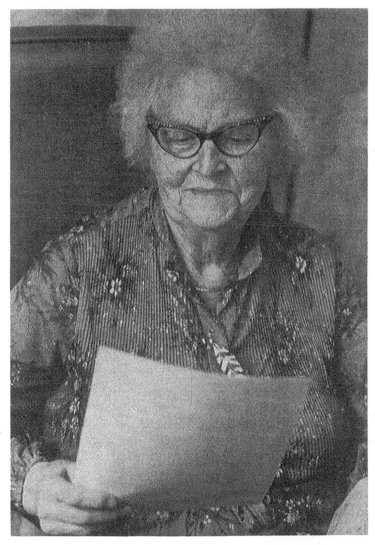

And poetry is an especially good activity for sharing memories.

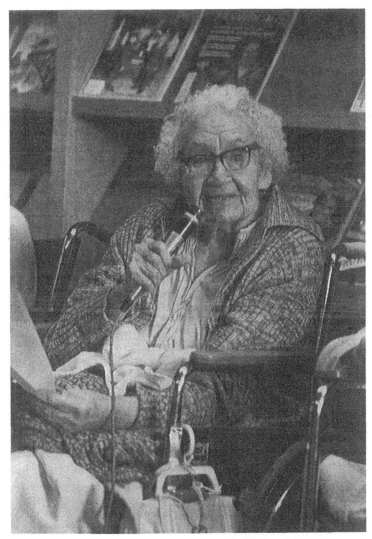

One of the most valued kinds of activities is one that a family member shares in with their elder. That may be in a group activity planned by the facility, or one which has special individualized meaning for the elder and family member.

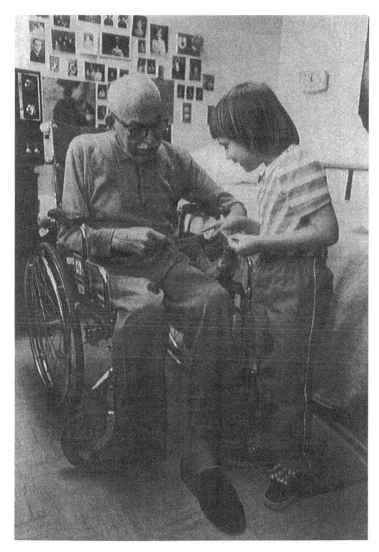

And along with opportunities for elders to receive special gifts and considerations,

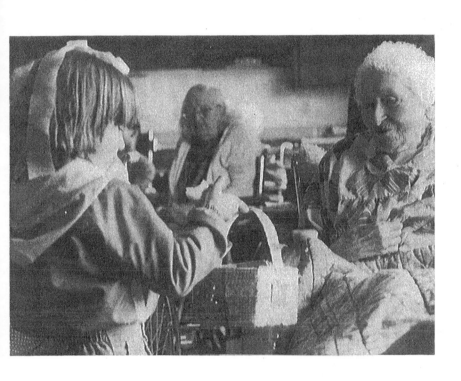

It is also important to plan events where the elders are not passive recipients, but are the ones on the giving end!

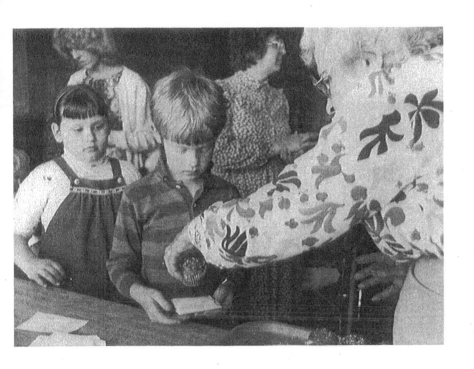

There is a more formal activity known as "Reality Orientation," where nursing home personnel or family members discuss current events and daily occurrences with the elder.

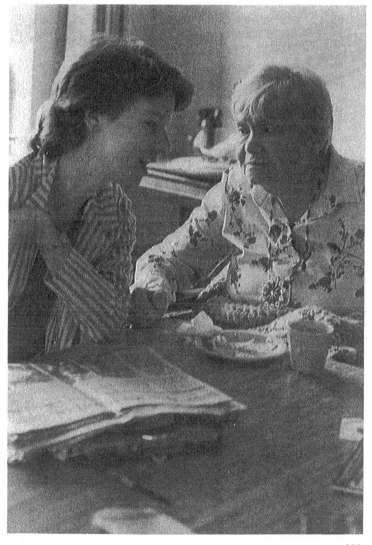

But the real value of Reality Orientation is not so much the reading of the newspaper, etc., but the opportunity for meaningful interaction.

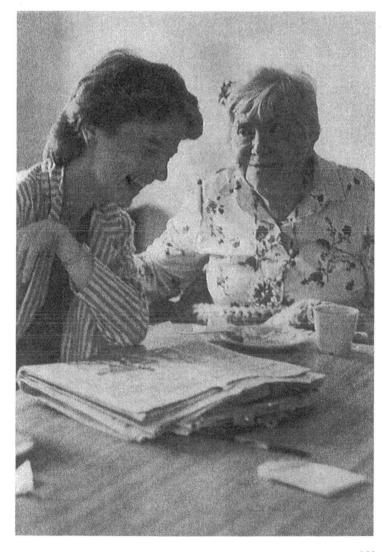

All this is not to imply activities must be goal oriented. A quiet visit with family may well be the most valued stimulation of all.

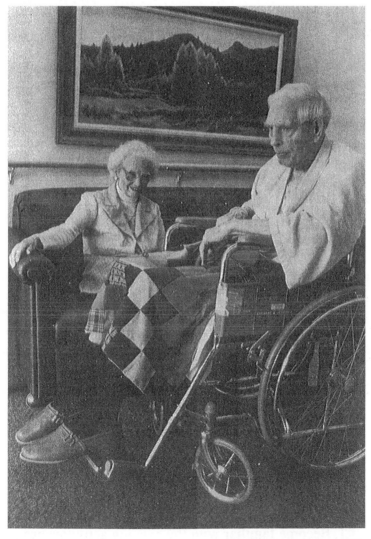

The guidelines that follow are for families caring for their elder's mental needs.

CHECKPOINT: DIFFERENTIATING BETWEEN "DIVERSIONARY ACTIVITIES" AND THOSE WHICH ENCOURAGE WHOLISTIC, CREATIVE GROWTH

There is a vast difference between activities which are designed as time-fillers to combat boredom and those which are designed to challenge the hearts and minds of elders, facilitating ongoing growth, self-appreciation, and self-knowledge.

Concern:

The concern is the issue of quantity vs. quality. There are numerous activities that can be done with elders to simply pass time. While it is true such activities combat boredom, they place the elder in the position of a child who must be entertained or put through its tricks and patted on the head. Activities which do not challenge the productive and uniquely creative abilities of the elder, nor impart any sense of inner worth miss the point of what an activity program is meant to be about.

Although there is a place for busy work, games, and talking "at" elders, an activities program built totally around such an approach neglects the dignity of elders and misses a critical opportunity for providing a climate of growth necessary for mental health.

What Do I Do?

1. Become familiar with the existing activities program and determine if there is a noticeable lack in this regard.

2. Read the resource material available which presents models of viable activities programs. Share what is possible with the activity director and administration. Much ineptness is directly related to being uninformed.
3. Engage on a one-to-one activities program with your elder, emphasizing activities which foster creative growth and wholistic productivity.

CHECKPOINT:
PERSONALIZING ACTIVITIES

The need for personalizing activities comes from the realization that there are a number of ways family members can design an activities program which can then become an integral part of their visiting: in essence, a program to supplement the nursing home's program.

Concern:

It is important to emphasize continually that stimulation appears to be the single most important factor mediating against withdrawal, disinterest, and psycho/social death (wherein a person simply gives up, and their death cannot be traced to organ pathology but seems more rooted in boredom and/or lack of meaning).

What Do I Do?

1. Give consideration to the types of activities your elder may have enjoyed prior to institutionalization; reading, gardening, sewing, whittling, writing? This information should also be supplied to the staff and activities personnel.
2. Work innovatively to recapture some of those interests, even though they have to be on an entirely different scale.

IDEAS FOR STARTERS:
Planting bulbs and seeds in pots rather than in a garden,
sprouting seeds like alfalfa and mung beans that grow
visibly every day and can be eaten in salads on meal trays
and shared with other elders.
Craft work—in particular making presents for grand-
children, children and special friends. Beads threaded for
necklaces (good physical therapy for finger manip-
ulation), collages from family photographic collections
which can then be framed; appliques for handkerchiefs
or scarves, painting material such as scarves with tube
paint; woodwork or gluing together pre-cut pieces to
form boxes, candle holders, etc.; any kind of knitting or
crocheting when applicable. Creative work: writing
stories, poems or songs together; making Christmas
cards, valentines, holiday favors.

CHECKPOINT:
REALITY ORIENTATION

Days seem to blend into one another when sitting or lying
day after day in a controlled environment. Time may appear
to stand still; memories can replace here-now awareness. If
the world appears to have come to a halt, so then does one's
perception of it. Reality Orientation is a form of stimulation
designed each day to focus the elder on the immediacies of
his/her life. Queries are put forth regarding one's name, one's
age, the date, the weather, and other issues designed to help
the elder focus on their immediate environment.

Concern:

Reality Orientation is usually under the direction of the activities director. However, for it to be effective, it needs to go
on throughout the day, rather than during just one time seg-

ment. For that reason, nursing assistants should be given in-service training in Reality Orientation as well as activities personnel. Much depends in this regard on the commitment of the nursing home. There is a growing concern about the lack of *ongoing consistent* Reality Orientation.

What Do I Do?

1. Sit in on Reality Orientation sessions conducted by activities personnel so you will understand how to participate in it yourself.
2. At the beginning, ending or some time during each visit with your elder, focus on Reality Orientation.
3. Encourage in-service programs in the nursing home for both family and nursing assistants wherein all parties can learn to appreciate the critical role of this activity and incorporate it into interactions with elders.

CHECKPOINT: REMOTIVATIONAL THERAPY

Remotivation is a technique of very simple group therapy which can be used by families as well as nurses, staff, and volunteers to reach the meaningful areas of an elder's personality. Its goal is to make reality a pleasant experience and to restore an elder's sense of worth.

Concern:

Much concern with elders in homes is superficial or patronizing. Remotivational Therapy is a skill that draws the elder into a discussion that will stimulate the motivating life experiences that are mentally pleasurable and emotionally uplifting. It is designed to establish in the elder a sense of personal worth and competency by giving them attention, and by recognizing them as persons who have knowledge and experiences that are both interesting and worth sharing with another.

What Do I Do?

1. Greet the elder cheerfully by name, saying something positive and honest. This is the first step of building a climate of acceptance.
2. Bring with you a news article, a picture from a magazine, a short, descriptive poem, or an object from home or the outside world for the second step which has to do with building a bridge to reality. The object must be something that appeals to the elder's sense of hearing, sight, taste, touch or smell.
3. Draw the elder out about what s/he knows about the nature of things. This is a way of exercising an unwounded area of their lives and allowing them to explore the world. Ask about their personal likes, about historical events and experiences.
4. Encourage the elder to share the work they have done. "How did you make pumpkin pie?" "How did you thresh the wheat?" It gives persons a sense of worth to share information and knowledge with another.
5. Remotivational Therapy always ends with gestures of appreciation: letting the elder know through word, touch or smile that being with them was interesting and enjoyable.

CHECKPOINT:
RESIDENT COUNCILS

Resident Councils are an effective way for elders to verbalize their concerns openly and participate in policies of the home which are directly related to their care.

Concern:

There is always the possibility that other considerations will take precedence over patients' rights; also because homes tend to function in parental ways, often overlooked is the fact that elders have clear and penetrating insights and need to be an integral part of the home's policy making.

What Do I Do?

1. Familiarize yourself with the Patient's Bill of Rights (see appendix).
2. Find out if the home has a Resident Council, and if so, is it truly vital and functioning? You can determine that by dialoguing with Resident Council members, reviewing the written record of their meetings, and in sitting in as observer/participants in their meetings.
3. Review the functions of a well-run and effective Resident Council:
   a. Making input into the development of the home's policies, especially those pertaining directly or indirectly to resident care.
   b. Making input into the inspection process of the State Health Division, especially in helping determine how well the home meets state and federal standards. Inspectors should be authorized to discuss points of investigation with Resident Councils.
   c. Participating in the development of public education programs. The intent here is to educate the public about nursing homes and nursing home life. Topics could include: "What is it like to live in a nursing home?" "How can nursing home residents be involved in the community?", etc.
   d. Guidelines for Resident Councils:
      —Council members should be elected by residents.

—The social worker or activities director should serve as the liaison between the council and the administration.

—The council should include a member of a resident's family or an interested party from the community.

—Meetings should be open to all interested parties and held on a regular basis.

4. If such a council is not functional, find out why.

If it is a matter of oversight, a delegation of residents should be encouraged to meet with staff and administration to gain support. Technical assistance for setting up councils can be obtained from local nursing home coalition groups: Gray Panther organizations, local agencies on aging, etc. The American Health Care Association has gone on record encouraging its members to develop resident councils.

If a viable resident council is *not* functioning because of home policy, one would question whether there is a true commitment to quality and democratic care and whether this is the best home for your elder.

CHECKPOINT:
FAMILY & FRIENDS COUNCILS

The whole intent of this manual is to show how vital a link family and friends are in nursing home care. Establishing a Family & Friends Council is an excellent way for families to combine interest, supportiveness and effort. In this way they conjointly become an effective coalition and can increase the effectiveness of the home. Further, such councils have a beneficial effect upon the morale of elders, nursing home staff and other families and friends.

Concern:

Families are closest to their elders if they visit frequently. They are more aware of the specific care needs than impersonal care-takers can be. Yet, often family members feel awkward and do not understand their rights and responsibilities in participating more fully within the structure of the home.

What Do I Do?

1. Understand the goals and objectives of Family & Friends Councils:
   a. Offering support to residents, helping with adjustment problems, helping to promote maximum functioning.
   b. Seeking to enhance public awareness of the problems and accomplishments of nursing homes and their residents.
   c. Helping families play a more vital role in meeting the personal needs of elders.
   d. Providing opportunities for family and friends to participate in policies affecting resident care.
   e. Promoting the Patient Bill of Rights.
2. Becoming aware of activities in which Family & Friends might participate:
   a. Fund raising for special projects in the home.
   b. Educating residents and family about the Patient Bill of Rights.
   c. Meeting with administrators and other nursing home personnel to discuss policies and make recommendations.
   d. Inspecting on a regular basis the survey reports of the State Health Division.

    e. Establishing support groups for residents and families in times of stress, crises and transition.

    f. Developing informational services for new residents and their family members.

    g. Participating in group activities for and with residents.

3. Starting a Family & Friends Council if none is currently in existence.

    a. Informally discuss the idea with other family members and friends you meet in the home to determine if there is an interest in forming a council.

    b. Schedule a meeting with the administrator of the home to enlist his/her support.

    c. Schedule a meeting for interested parties, having a clear understanding of the goals and objectives.

    d. Maintain frequent communication, participating as fully as possible in nursing home life at all levels.

NOTE: It takes effort to establish a Family & Friends Council. If you have the cooperation of the nursing home, it is much easier. If you do not, the Council must work very creatively to be a viable source of support for the residents.

HOW TO CARE FOR, COMFORT, AND COMMUNE AT THE SPIRITUAL LEVEL

Care and comfort of the Spirit are of particular importance to many institutionalized elders no longer able to attend church. Nursing homes generally offer non-denominational worship services for those who wish to attend.

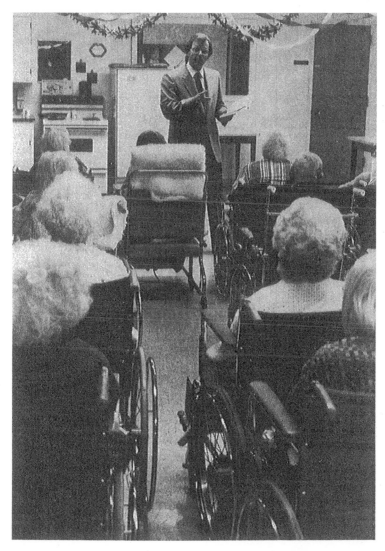

But mostly the spiritual needs of those nearing the close of life are personal and private. Meaningful prayer and bible study cannot be placed on an activities schedule. They need to be honored in quiet with loved ones.

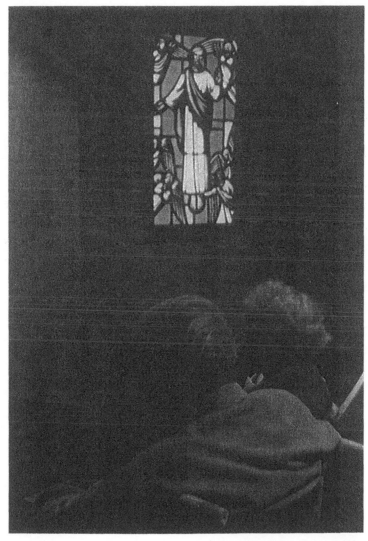

If a formal place of worship is unavailable, togetherness in an area removed from noise and distraction is sufficient. The atmosphere becomes peaceful through reflection and worship.

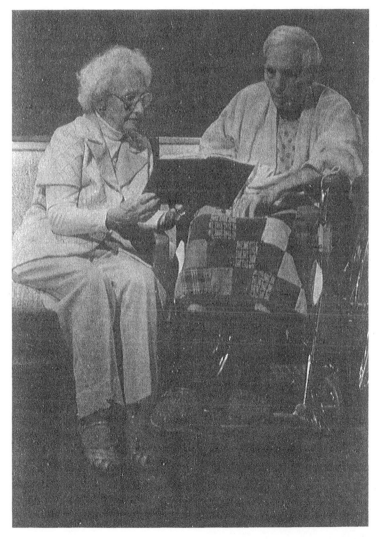

Ultimately, death must be confronted by the elder; by the family. And as misunderstood as death may be, it does somehow affirm the meaning of life. A meaning that may well depend on how we have chosen to respond to life's challenges; none the least of which being how we have loved.

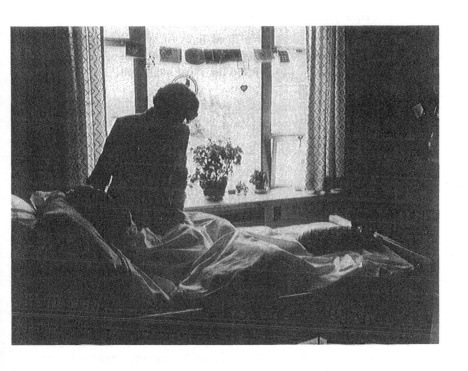

The guidelines that follow are for families caring for their elder's spiritual needs.

CHECKPOINT:
SPECIAL TIMES FOR SPIRITUAL LIFE

Many of our elders have lived lives of spiritual commitment. If they are not able to be placed in a church sponsored home, this area of life is often the most neglected.

Concern:

Most nursing homes do not have chapels or rooms for quiet, spiritual reflection. Some type of weekly service is offered, including prayers and hymns, but most are modeled on parent-child relationships: i.e. doing the service for elders rather than with them. How much more sensitive when elders are encouraged to speak and share their faith.

What Do I Do?

1. Find out what the personal spiritual needs are of your family member. Do they involve saying grace before meals, reading the Bible aloud or hearing it read aloud, devotional study, hearing favorite hymns or singing them with others? How can you participate in sharing and helping fulfill those needs on an ongoing basis?
2. Encourage the formulation of an activities program that acknowledges and enhances the spiritual life of elders. This could take the form of small prayer groups, Bible discussion groups, faith healing for one another. Families can be instrumental in taking the lead in these kinds of programs, particularly on Sunday when activities are less planned.

CHECKPOINT:
VISITS FROM CHURCH MEMBERS,
MINISTERS, PRIESTS?

Visitors are always a welcome treat for those in nursing homes, particularly when from the church which has been an integral part of an elder's life.

Concern:

Churches need to be informed of living arrangements so they can work out schedules of visiting and communion.

What Do I Do?

1. Notify the church when an elder is placed in a nursing home. Request visits and communion.
2. Let the church know the better time for visiting when your elder is most apt to be up and in a position for receiving visitors. It is a great disappointment to awaken from an afternoon nap only to find a visiting card left on the nightstand.
3. Make arrangements to be on hand if possible when communion is brought. Sharing sacraments can be a very deep source of caring and interaction.

CHECKPOINT:
PREPARING FOR DEATH

Death is a familiar visitor to nursing homes, but not one often talked about. Many elders have come to a quiet acceptance of death; others harbor fears and unresolved conflicts.

Concern:

Persons die in nursing homes but are not *prepared* for death in nursing homes. If it is difficult for family or staff to deal openly with their own death fears, it is impossible to lend support to an elder at this transitional state.

What Do I Do?

1. First confront your own fears about death and dying. "Thanatology" is a new term for the study of death. Workshops and classes are being conducted throughout the country to enable persons to more comfortably confront the issues involved in death and dying. A wide range of source material is available for reading.
2. Give consideration to any unfinished business you have with your family member. Many persons suffer from intense guilt after the death of a relative, remembering what they neglected to say or do for that person.
3. Once you feel on terms with your own death, you are ready to help your elder with any issues surrounding their own which are yet to be dealt with.

   Various kinds of creative work can be done in this regard. Ruby Miller, to whom this book is dedicated, wrote a poem about her death which she requested have read at her funeral.

   Having persons draw their conception of death is a powerful way of sharing the feeling one has connected to the dying process. It also facilitates communication, as so many persons find it difficult to speak openly about their feelings regarding death.

   Often dream content reflects death concerns that are not able to be verbalized in other ways. There is always a place for sharing dreams and using them as a means of deeper communication.

   Are there special things your elder would like to do prior to death? Letters to friends, a visit by telephone with family members they have not seen for some time?

   Be extremely sensitive to the needs of the last months and

years of your elder. Perhaps the ultimate form of helpmating is allowing a loved one to die in peace (although it may not be a painless peace), knowing their life has found meaningful closure.

IN CONCLUSION

This book has been about care giving. It has assumed families—some families—will want to give care in a most total way.

The guidelines have been suggested in full knowledge that such care is demanding, exhausting, and emotionally tearing. Yet, there will always be those who respond: "Why not? What else has meaning?"

They are the ones for whom this book has been written. Ironically, they are not those who need guidelines. Their care is unconditional; therefore complete. Complete whether guidelines for care are followed or not.

So if this author is presumptious in cook-booking care, she knows the readers will be tolerant. Both she and they know love cannot be categorized.

Love gives of itself in ways that will not be reduced to formulas. And love keeps on giving because it knows no other way.

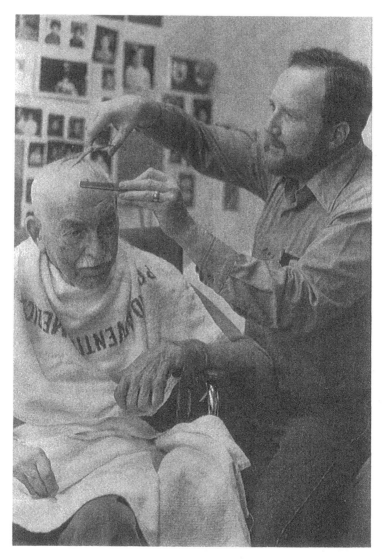

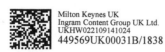